HOW TO LOSS WEIGHT FAST: 4 SIMPLE STRATEGY TO EFFECTIVE WEIGHT LOSS IN 7 DAYS

CELESTINE BENEDICT

DEDICATION

To my beloved parents, who have always encouraged me to chase my dreams and to never give up on my passions. Your love and support have been the foundation of my success and have helped me to reach new heights. This book is dedicated to you, with gratitude for all that you have done and for being my biggest fans.

And to all those who are striving to achieve their health and wellness goals, this book is for you. May it serve as a guide and inspiration as you embark on your journey towards a healthier and happier life.

TABLE OF CONTENTS

How to loss weight fast.

ACKNOWLEDGMENTS

First and foremost, I would like to express my heartfelt gratitude to my family and friends who have been my constant source of inspiration and support throughout my journey of writing this book. Your unwavering belief in me and my abilities has been a driving force behind my passion and commitment to this project.

I am deeply grateful to all the experts and professionals in the field of health and wellness who have generously shared their knowledge and expertise with me. Your invaluable insights and advice have been instrumental in shaping the content of this book and providing readers with practical and actionable steps for losing weight fast.

Finally, I would like to thank my readers for choosing to pick up this book. I hope that you find the information and guidance within these pages to be helpful and empowering as you work towards achieving your health and wellness goals.

CHAPTER ONE

INTRODUCTION

OVERVIEW OF THIS BOOK

Losing weight can be a challenging task for many people, but with the right approach, it can be an achievable goal. This book, "How to Lose Weight Fast: 4 Simple Strategies for Effective Weight Loss," provides a comprehensive guide for those looking to shed excess pounds and improve their overall health and well-being. The book outlines four simple strategies that, when combined and implemented consistently, can help individuals reach their weight loss goals effectively and sustainably.

This book is designed to provide readers with a comprehensive and straightforward guide to weight loss. The first section of the book provides an overview of the importance of weight loss and the four simple strategies that will be covered in the following chapters. The remaining chapters delve into each of the four strategies in detail, explaining the science behind them, offering practical tips and advice, and providing examples to help readers put the strategies into practice.

The four strategies covered in the book are:

Implementing a healthy diet
Engaging in regular physical activity
Managing stress and sleep habits
Staying motivated and on track

Each of these strategies plays a critical role in the weight loss process, and the book provides readers with the tools and information they need to successfully integrate them into their daily lives. The book also provides practical tips and advice to help readers overcome common challenges and obstacles that can arise during the weight loss journey.

IMPORTANCE OF WEIGHT LOSS

Weight loss is important for a number of reasons, including improved overall health, increased energy levels, reduced risk of chronic diseases, and improved self-esteem and body image. Maintaining a healthy weight can also help individuals lead longer, more fulfilling lives.

However, weight loss can also be challenging, and many people struggle to achieve their goals. This is where the strategies outlined in this book can help. By providing a comprehensive and evidence-based approach to weight loss, this book can help individuals achieve their goals and make the process of weight loss more manageable and sustainable.

Weight loss is a critical aspect of overall health and well-being, and has numerous benefits that can improve an individual's quality of life. From reducing the risk of chronic diseases to improving self-esteem and body image, the importance of weight loss cannot be overstated.

Reduced Risk of Chronic Diseases

Excess weight can increase the risk of a number of chronic diseases, including heart disease, diabetes, and certain cancers. By losing weight and maintaining a healthy weight, individuals can reduce their risk of developing these chronic diseases and improve their overall health and longevity.

Improved Energy Levels

Being overweight or obese can make it difficult to engage in physical activity, and can lead to feelings of fatigue and low energy levels. By losing weight and engaging in regular physical activity, individuals can experience improved energy levels, making it easier to participate in daily activities and lead a more active, fulfilling life.

Improved Self-Esteem and Body Image

Excess weight can have a significant impact on an individual's self-esteem and body image. By losing weight, individuals can improve their confidence and self-esteem, leading to improved overall well-being and quality of life.

Reduced Risk of Depression and Anxiety

Studies have shown that individuals who are overweight or obese are at an increased risk of depression and anxiety. By losing weight, individuals can reduce this risk and improve their overall mental health and well-being.

Improved Cardiovascular Health

Excess weight can increase the risk of heart disease, high blood pressure, and stroke. By losing weight and maintaining a healthy weight, individuals can improve their cardiovascular health, reducing their risk of heart disease and other cardiovascular conditions.

Improved Mobility and Flexibility

Excess weight can make it difficult to engage in physical activity and can lead to joint pain and mobility problems. By losing weight, individuals can improve their mobility and flexibility, making it easier to engage in physical activity and lead an active, fulfilling life.

Weight loss is an important aspect of overall health and well-being, with numerous benefits that can improve an individual's quality of life. From reducing the risk of chronic diseases to improving self-esteem and body image, the importance of weight loss cannot be overstated. By making changes to their diet and lifestyle and adopting a comprehensive weight loss strategy, individuals can achieve their weight loss goals and lead healthier, more fulfilling lives.

UNDERSTANDING THE 4 SIMPLE STRATEGIES

The four simple strategies outlined in this book have been carefully selected and are based on the latest scientific research on weight loss. They have been proven to be effective in helping individuals achieve their weight loss goals and maintain a healthy weight in the long-term.

Implementing a healthy diet, engaging in regular physical

activity, managing stress and sleep habits, and staying motivated and on track are all critical components of a successful weight loss journey. The book provides readers with the tools and information they need to understand and effectively implement each of these strategies in their daily lives.

The book, "How to Lose Weight Fast: 4 Simple Strategies for Effective Weight Loss," is a comprehensive guide for those looking to lose weight and improve their overall health and well-being. The four simple strategies outlined in the book have been carefully selected and are based on the latest scientific research on weight loss. By providing a clear and practical guide to weight loss, this book can help individuals achieve their goals and lead healthier, more fulfilling lives.

CHAPTER TWO

STRATEGY 1

IMPLEMENTING A HEALTHY DIET

The first strategy for weight loss is to implement a healthy diet. This involves understanding the concept of caloric balance, identifying healthy food choices, and incorporating meal planning and preparation techniques into your routine. Caloric balance refers to the relationship between the number of calories you consume and the number of calories you burn through physical activity. To lose weight, you need to create a caloric deficit by consuming fewer calories than you burn.

When it comes to food choices, it's important to focus on nutrient-dense, whole foods, such as fruits and vegetables, lean proteins, and whole grains. These foods will help you feel full and satisfied, while also providing the nutrients your body needs to function optimally.

Meal planning and preparation can also play a crucial role in weight loss success. By planning and preparing your meals ahead of time, you can ensure that you have healthy options readily available and avoid making unhealthy choices when you're short on time.

UNDERSTANDING CALORIC BALANCE

Caloric balance is a crucial concept in weight loss and weight management. It refers to the relationship between the number of calories you consume and the number of calories you burn through physical activity. By understanding the concept of caloric balance, you can take control of your weight and reach your health and fitness goals.

What is Caloric Balance?

Caloric balance is a simple equation: the number of calories you consume must either equal or be less than the number of calories you burn in order to lose weight. If you consume more calories than you burn, you will gain weight. Conversely, if you consume fewer calories than you burn, you will lose weight.

The number of calories you need to consume depends on several factors, including your age, gender, height, weight, and level of physical activity. A sedentary person who does not engage in physical activity will require fewer calories than someone who is highly active.

The number of calories you burn depends on your basal metabolic rate (BMR), which is the amount of energy your body needs to function at rest, and your level of physical activity. Your BMR accounts for the majority of your daily energy expenditure, with physical activity and digestion accounting for the remaining energy expenditure.

The Importance of Caloric Balance for Weight Loss

Caloric balance is crucial for weight loss because it determines the number of calories you need to consume and the number of calories you need to burn in order to reach your weight loss goals. By creating a caloric deficit, you can effectively lose weight.

A caloric deficit can be achieved in several ways,

including reducing the number of calories you consume, increasing the number of calories you burn through physical activity, or a combination of both. It's important to remember that weight loss is a slow process and that it's not recommended to create a caloric deficit of more than 500-1000 calories per day.

Creating a caloric deficit requires a healthy and balanced diet that includes a variety of nutrient-dense foods, such as fruits and vegetables, lean proteins, and whole grains. It's also important to limit your intake of processed foods and added sugars, which are high in calories and low in nutrients.

Incorporating physical activity into your routine is another effective way to create a caloric deficit and reach your weight loss goals. Regular physical activity can boost your metabolism, increase the number of calories you burn, and improve your overall health and fitness. It's recommended that you engage in at least 150 minutes of moderate-intensity physical activity or 75 minutes of vigorous-intensity physical activity per week.

The Benefits of Understanding Caloric Balance

Understanding caloric balance provides several benefits, including:

- Improved weight management: By understanding the relationship between the number of calories you consume and the number of calories you burn, you can take control of your weight and reach your weight loss goals.

- Better nutrition: By focusing on nutrient-dense foods and limiting your intake of processed foods and added sugars, you can improve your overall nutrition and support good health.

- Increased physical activity: By incorporating physical activity into your routine, you can increase the number of calories you burn, improve your overall health and fitness, and support weight loss.

- Improved health: By achieving a healthy weight and improving your nutrition and physical activity habits, you can reduce your risk of chronic diseases, such as heart disease, stroke, and type 2 diabetes

The concept of caloric balance is a simple equation that is crucial for weight loss and weight management. By understanding the relationship between the number of calories you consume and the number of calories you burn, you can take control of your weight and reach your health and fitness goals.

IDENTIFYING HEALTHY FOOD CHOICES

Identifying healthy food choices is an important aspect of weight management and overall health. Making smart food choices is crucial for creating a caloric deficit, which is necessary for weight loss, and for obtaining the nutrients your body needs to function optimally.

Healthy food choices include nutrient-dense foods that provide your body with essential vitamins, minerals, and fiber, while being low in calories and unhealthy fats. Some examples of healthy food choices include fruits and vegetables, whole grains, lean proteins, and healthy fats.

Fruits and Vegetables

Fruits and vegetables are excellent sources of vitamins, minerals, and fiber. They are also low in calories, making them ideal for weight management. Eating a variety of colorful fruits and vegetables provides your body with a wide range of nutrients and helps to prevent nutrient deficiencies.

Some examples of nutrient-dense fruits and vegetables include leafy greens, such as kale and spinach, brightly colored fruits and vegetables, such as blueberries and bell peppers, and cruciferous vegetables, such as broccoli and cauliflower.

Whole Grains

Whole grains are an excellent source of fiber and other

important nutrients, including B vitamins, iron, and magnesium. Unlike refined grains, whole grains contain all parts of the grain, including the bran, germ, and endosperm, which provides your body with essential nutrients and fiber.

Examples of whole grains include brown rice, quinoa, whole-grain bread and pasta, and whole-grain cereal. It's important to choose whole grain options instead of refined grain options, as refined grains have been stripped of essential nutrients and fiber.

Lean Proteins

Lean proteins are an important component of a healthy diet, as they provide your body with essential amino acids and help to build and repair tissues. Lean protein sources are low in unhealthy fats and calories, making them ideal for weight management.

Examples of lean protein sources include chicken, turkey, fish, tofu, and legumes. It's important to vary your protein sources, as each type of protein provides your body with different nutrients and benefits.

Healthy Fats

Healthy fats are an essential component of a healthy diet, as they provide your body with energy and help to absorb fat-soluble vitamins. Healthy fats also help to improve heart health, reduce inflammation, and support brain function.

Examples of healthy fats include avocado, nuts, seeds, olive oil, and fatty fish, such as salmon. It's important to limit your intake of unhealthy fats, such as trans fats and saturated fats, as these types of fats can increase your risk of heart disease and other chronic health conditions.

Foods to Avoid

In addition to identifying healthy food choices, it's also important to limit or avoid certain types of foods that are high in calories, unhealthy fats, and added sugars. Some examples of foods to limit or avoid include:

- Processed Foods: Processed foods are often high in calories, unhealthy fats, and added sugars, and low in essential nutrients. Examples of processed foods include snack foods, such as chips and crackers, and convenience foods, such as frozen dinners and packaged snacks.

- Added Sugars: Added sugars are often found in sweetened beverages, such as soda and fruit juice, and in sweets, such as candy and baked goods. These types of foods are high in calories and low in essential nutrients, making them a poor choice for weight management.

- Unhealthy Fats: Unhealthy fats, such as trans fats and saturated fats, can increase your risk of heart disease and other chronic health conditions. Examples of foods high in unhealthy fats include fried foods, such as french fries and fried chicken, and foods.

MEAL PLANNING AND PREPARATION TECHNIQUES

One of the keys to a successful weight loss journey is eating a healthy, balanced diet. Meal planning and preparation can help you achieve your weight loss goals by ensuring that you have healthy, nutritious food available when you need it. In this section, we will discuss practical tips and techniques for meal planning and preparation that can help you achieve your weight loss goals.

- Plan Your Meals: The first step in successful meal planning and preparation is to plan your meals. Consider using a meal planning app or writing out a weekly menu to help you stay organized. Make sure to include a variety of healthy foods, such as fruits, vegetables, whole grains, and lean protein, in your meal plan.

- Make a Grocery List: Once you have planned your meals, make a grocery list of the ingredients you need. This will help you stay focused while shopping and ensure that you have everything you need to prepare healthy, nutritious meals.

- Shop for Healthy Ingredients: When shopping for ingredients, make sure to choose healthy, whole foods. Look for fresh fruits and vegetables, whole grains, lean protein, and healthy fats. Avoid processed foods and foods high in sugar and unhealthy fats.

- Cook in Bulk: Cooking in bulk can save you time and money, and it also makes it easier to have healthy, nutritious food available when you need it. Consider cooking larger portions of healthy meals and storing leftovers in the refrigerator or freezer for later.

- Use a Slow Cooker: A slow cooker can be a great tool for meal planning and preparation. Consider using a slow cooker to prepare healthy stews, soups, and casseroles that can be eaten throughout the week.

- Try Meal Prepping: Meal prepping, or preparing multiple meals at once, can be a great way to save time and stay on track with your weight loss goals. Consider preparing several portions of healthy meals in advance and storing them in the refrigerator or freezer for later.

- Make Healthy Snacks: In addition to meal planning and preparation, it is important to have healthy snacks available when you need them. Consider making your own healthy snacks, such as trail mix, fresh fruit, or hummus and vegetables, to have on hand.

- Avoid Eating Out: Eating out at restaurants can be a major source of unhealthy food and excess calories. Consider cooking healthy meals at home and bringing them with you when you are on the go.

- Get Creative in the Kitchen: Cooking can be a fun and creative activity, and it is also an opportunity to try new recipes and ingredients. Consider trying new recipes and experimenting with healthy ingredients to find new and delicious ways to eat well.

- In conclusion, meal planning and preparation is an essential component of a successful weight loss plan. By planning your meals, shopping for healthy ingredients, cooking in bulk, using a slow cooker, meal prepping, making healthy snacks, avoiding eating out, and getting creative in the kitchen, you can achieve your weight loss goals and eat well along the way. With a little planning and effort, you can create a meal plan and preparation strategy that works for you and helps you achieve your weight loss goals

COMMON DIET MISTAKES TO AVOID: A GUIDE TO EFFECTIVE WEIGHT LOSS

When it comes to weight loss, many people make common mistakes that can hinder their progress. These mistakes can be as simple as not tracking your calorie intake or skipping meals, or as complicated as following fad diets or making unrealistic goals.

To achieve your weight loss goals and maintain a healthy lifestyle, it's important to avoid these common diet mistakes. Here are some of the most common diet mistakes and how to avoid them.

Skipping meals

One of the biggest mistakes people make when trying to lose weight is skipping meals. Skipping meals leads to overeating later in the day, which can cause weight gain. Skipping breakfast, in particular, can lead to overeating later in the day. Instead of skipping meals, try eating smaller, more frequent meals throughout the day to keep your metabolism going and prevent overeating.

Not tracking your calorie intake

It's important to know how many calories you are consuming and how many calories you are burning. Not tracking your calorie intake can cause you to consume more calories than you think, which can result in weight gain. Try using a food journal or an app to track your calorie intake and monitor your progress.

Fad diets

Fad diets promise quick weight loss, but they are not sustainable and often lead to weight gain in the long term. Fad diets can be harmful to your health and often restrict essential nutrients and foods. Instead of following fad diets, focus on making healthy food choices and incorporating physical activity into your daily routine.

Eliminating entire food groups

Eliminating entire food groups, such as carbohydrates or fat, can be harmful to your health and can lead to weight gain. Your body needs a balance of all macronutrients (carbohydrates, fat, and protein) to function properly. Instead of eliminating entire food groups, try to make healthier choices within each food group and aim for moderation.

Making unrealistic goals

Making unrealistic weight loss goals can be harmful to your mental and physical health. Rapid weight loss is not sustainable and often leads to weight gain in the long term. Set realistic goals and aim to lose weight slowly and steadily over time.

Eating too much processed and high-calorie food

Eating too much processed and high-calorie food can cause weight gain and harm your health. Processed foods often contain high amounts of sugar, salt, and unhealthy fats. Try to limit your consumption of processed and high-calorie food and make healthier food choices, such as fresh fruits and vegetables, lean protein, and whole grains.

Eating out too often

Eating out at restaurants can be tempting, but it can also be high in calories and unhealthy ingredients. Restaurant meals often contain large portions and unhealthy ingredients, such as high amounts of sugar, salt, and unhealthy fats. Try to limit your eating out to once or twice a week and make healthier choices when eating out.

Not drinking enough water

Drinking enough water is important for weight loss and overall health. Not drinking enough water can cause dehydration, which can lead to overeating and weight gain. Aim to drink at least 8 glasses of water a day and try to limit your consumption of sugary drinks, such as soda and juice.

CHAPTER THREE

STRATEGY 2

ENGAGING IN REGULAR PHYSICAL ACTIVITY

The second strategy for weight loss is to engage in regular physical activity. Exercise has numerous benefits, including boosting your metabolism, improving your mood, and helping you burn calories. To achieve the best results, it's recommended that you engage in a combination of cardiovascular exercise, such as running or cycling, and strength training, such as weight lifting or bodyweight exercises.

When determining your exercise routine, it's important to find activities that you enjoy and that you can realistically incorporate into your daily routine. This could be anything from going for a walk or jog to joining a gym or sports team. The key is to find something that you enjoy and can stick to.

TYPES OF PHYSICAL ACTIVITIES FOR WEIGHT LOSS

Physical activity is an essential component of a weight loss plan, and it can be helpful to understand the different types of activities that are available to you. Whether you are looking to increase your heart rate and burn calories, build muscle, or simply stay active, there is a type of physical activity that is right for you. Here are some of the most popular types of physical activities for weight loss:

Cardiovascular Exercise

Cardiovascular exercise is any form of exercise that raises your heart rate and helps improve your cardiovascular health. Examples of cardiovascular exercise include running, cycling, swimming, and jumping rope. Cardiovascular exercise is particularly effective for weight loss because it burns a lot of calories in a short period of time, making it an excellent way to lose weight quickly. Additionally, cardiovascular exercise can help increase your metabolism, making it easier for you to burn calories even when you are not working out.

Strength Training

Strength training is an effective way to build muscle, which helps increase metabolism and burn more calories even when you are not working out. Strength training can be done using weights or resistance bands, and it can be performed at home or in a gym. Strength training can help you build muscle, which is particularly important for people who are looking to lose weight, as muscle tissue burns more calories than fat tissue.

HIIT (High-Intensity Interval Training)

HIIT is a type of cardiovascular exercise that involves alternating between periods of high-intensity exercise and periods of rest. HIIT is an effective way to lose weight because it burns a lot of calories in a short period of time, and it also helps increase metabolism. Additionally, HIIT can be done using a variety of different exercises, making it a versatile form of exercise that is suitable for people of all fitness levels.

Yoga

Yoga is a form of exercise that involves stretching, holding poses, and focusing on breathing. Yoga can be a great form of exercise for weight loss because it helps increase flexibility, balance, and core strength, which can help you burn more calories during other forms of exercise. Additionally, yoga is a low-impact form of exercise, making it an excellent option for people who are looking to avoid high-impact exercises like running.

Dancing

Dancing is a fun and effective way to lose weight because it involves moving your entire body, which helps you burn calories and build muscle. Dancing can also be a great way to improve cardiovascular health and increase your overall fitness level. Whether you prefer ballroom dancing, hip-hop, or salsa, dancing can be a fun and effective way to lose weight and stay active.

Hiking

Hiking is a form of exercise that involves walking or trekking on rough terrain. Hiking can be a great form of exercise for weight loss because it involves a lot of leg and core muscles, which helps you burn a lot of calories in a short period of time. Additionally, hiking can help improve cardiovascular health, increase stamina, and reduce stress levels.

Swimming

Swimming is a great form of exercise for weight loss because it involves a lot of different muscles, which helps you burn a lot of calories in a short period of time. Swimming is also a low-impact form of exercise, making it an excellent option for people who are looking to avoid high-impact exercises like running. Additionally, swimming can help improve cardiovascular health, increase stamina, and reduce stress levels.

Sports

Playing sports is a fun and effective way to lose weight because it involves a lot of movement and physical activity. Whether you prefer basketball, soccer, tennis, or any other sport, playing sports can help you burn calories.

DETERMINING YOUR EXERCISE ROUTINE

When it comes to weight loss, engaging in regular physical activity is an essential component of a successful plan. However, with so many different types of physical activities available, it can be challenging to determine which exercise routine is right for you. In this section, we will discuss how to determine your exercise routine and make sure that it is effective and enjoyable.

Start by Assessing Your Current Fitness Level

Before you can determine your exercise routine, it is important to assess your current fitness level. This includes considering factors such as your age, health status, and any physical limitations you may have. This will help you understand what types of physical activities are suitable for you and which exercises you should avoid.

Set Realistic Goals

Once you have assessed your current fitness level, it is time to set realistic goals for your exercise routine. Consider what you want to achieve through your physical activity, whether it be weight loss, improved cardiovascular health, or simply staying active. Setting realistic goals will help you stay motivated and focused on your weight loss journey.

Choose a Type of Physical Activity That You Enjoy

When it comes to weight loss, consistency is key, and choosing a type of physical activity that you enjoy is an important part of staying motivated. Whether you prefer cardiovascular exercise, strength training, yoga, or any other form of physical activity, make sure that you choose a type of exercise that you enjoy and look forward to doing on a regular basis.

Make a Schedule

Once you have chosen a type of physical activity that you enjoy, it is time to make a schedule for your exercise routine. This includes determining how often you want to exercise and how long each session should last. Make sure that your schedule is realistic and takes into account any other commitments you may have.

Incorporate Variety

While it is important to have a consistent exercise routine, it is also important to incorporate variety into your routine to avoid boredom and maintain your interest. Consider trying different types of physical activities or mixing up your routine by combining different forms of exercise. This can help you stay motivated and engaged in your weight loss journey.

Work with a Personal Trainer

If you are new to exercise or have any physical limitations, working with a personal trainer can be a great way to determine your exercise routine. A personal trainer can help you assess your fitness level, set realistic goals, and develop a customized exercise plan that is tailored to your needs and abilities.

Gradually Increase Intensity

Once you have established a consistent exercise routine, it is important to gradually increase the intensity of your physical activity. This can include increasing the duration of your workouts, adding weights or resistance bands to your strength training routine, or increasing the difficulty of your yoga poses. Gradually increasing intensity will help you avoid injury and achieve your weight loss goals more quickly.

Determining your exercise routine is an important part of a successful weight loss plan. By assessing your current fitness level, setting realistic goals, choosing a type of physical activity that you enjoy, making a schedule, and gradually increasing intensity, you can ensure that your exercise routine is effective and enjoyable. Remember, consistency is key, and by making physical activity a regular part of your life, you will be on your way to achieving your weight loss goals

INCORPORATING PHYSICAL ACTIVITY INTO YOUR DAILY ROUTINE

Physical activity is an essential component of a successful weight loss plan, but it can be challenging to incorporate regular exercise into your daily routine. In this section, we will discuss practical tips and strategies for making physical activity a regular part of your life.

#Make Exercise a Priority

To successfully incorporate physical activity into your daily routine, it is important to make exercise a priority. This means setting aside time each day specifically for physical activity and making sure that it is a non-negotiable part of your daily schedule.

#Start Small

If you are new to exercise or are having trouble making physical activity a regular part of your routine, start small. Begin by incorporating short bouts of physical activity into your day, such as taking a 10-minute walk during your lunch break or doing a few minutes of stretching before bed. As you become more comfortable with exercise, you can gradually increase the duration and intensity of your physical activity.

#Find an Exercise Partner

Having an exercise partner can be a great way to stay motivated and accountable. Consider finding a workout buddy or joining a fitness group to help you stay on track with your exercise routine.

#Make Exercise Fun

Incorporating physical activity into your daily routine is much easier when you find an activity that you enjoy. Consider trying different types of physical activity until you find one that you look forward to doing on a regular basis. Whether it is dancing, swimming, or playing a sport, making exercise fun will help you stay motivated and engaged in your weight loss journey.

#Incorporate Physical Activity into Your Commute

If you have a sedentary job or spend a lot of time sitting throughout the day, incorporating physical activity into your daily routine can be challenging. One solution is to incorporate physical activity into your commute. Consider taking public transportation and walking or biking to work instead of driving, or take the stairs instead of the elevator.

#Use Technology

Technology can be a great tool for helping you incorporate physical activity into your daily routine. Consider using a fitness tracker to monitor your physical activity and set daily goals, or use a mobile app to find new and interesting workouts to try.

Schedule Exercise Time

Scheduling time for physical activity is an important part of making it a regular part of your routine. Consider scheduling a set time each day for exercise, such as a morning workout or a lunchtime walk. By making exercise a scheduled part of your day, you are more likely to stick with it and see results.

Be Creative

There are many ways to incorporate physical activity into your daily routine, and being creative can help you find new and interesting ways to stay active. Consider trying new physical activities, such as rock climbing, kayaking, or stand-up paddleboarding, or find creative ways to integrate physical activity into your daily life, such as doing household chores or gardening.

Make Exercise a Family Affair

Incorporating physical activity into your daily routine can be easier when you make it a family affair. Consider finding physical activities that you can do with your spouse, children, or friends, such as hiking, playing sports, or taking dance classes.

In conclusion, incorporating physical activity into your daily routine is an important part of a successful weight loss plan. By making exercise a priority, starting small, finding an exercise partner, making exercise fun, and incorporating physical activity into your daily life, you can successfully make physical activity a regular part of your life and achieve your weight loss goals. With a little creativity and determination, you can make physical activity a fun and enjoyable part of your daily routine.

CHAPTER FOUR

STRATEGY 3

MANAGING STRESS AND SLEEEP HABIT

The Impact of Stress on Weight Loss

Stress can have a significant impact on weight loss and overall health. Chronic stress can lead to hormonal imbalances, unhealthy coping mechanisms such as overeating, and a lack of motivation to engage in physical activity. Understanding the impact of stress on weight loss can help you develop effective strategies for managing stress and achieving your weight loss goals.

Hormonal Imbalances

Chronic stress can cause hormonal imbalances that can make it difficult to lose weight. The hormone cortisol, which is released in response to stress, can cause an increase in appetite and lead to overeating and weight gain. Cortisol also decreases insulin sensitivity, which can make it harder to regulate blood sugar levels and control cravings.

Unhealthy Coping Mechanisms

Stress can also lead to unhealthy coping mechanisms, such as overeating or binge eating, that can sabotage weight loss efforts. Comfort eating is a common way for people to cope with stress, but it can lead to weight gain and other health problems.

Lack of Motivation

Stress can also sap motivation and make it difficult to stick to a weight loss plan. When you are feeling stressed and overwhelmed, it can be hard to find the energy and motivation to engage in physical activity and make healthy food choices.

Sleep Deprivation

Stress can also cause sleep deprivation, which can impact weight loss and overall health. When you are not getting enough sleep, it can be harder to control cravings, maintain energy levels, and stick to a healthy eating plan.

Decreased Metabolism

Chronic stress can also slow down your metabolism, making it harder to lose weight. This can be due to the effects of cortisol on the body, which can slow down the metabolism and make it harder to burn fat.

In order to minimize the impact of stress on weight loss, it is important to develop effective strategies for managing stress. Consider the following tips:

Tip 1
Practice Mindfulness

Mindfulness practices, such as meditation and yoga, can help reduce stress and promote relaxation. By focusing on the present moment, mindfulness can help you reduce anxiety and feel more relaxed.

Tip 2
Exercise Regularly

Regular exercise is a great way to relieve stress and boost mood. Exercise releases endorphins, which are the body's natural feel-good chemicals, and it can help reduce anxiety and stress levels.

Tip 3
Get Enough Sleep

Sleep is important for overall health, including weight loss. Aim to get 7-8 hours of sleep each night and make sure to avoid late-night snacking and caffeine consumption before bed.

Tip 4
Connect with Others

Spending time with friends and family can help relieve stress and promote relaxation. Consider joining a support group or taking part in social activities that you enjoy.

Tip 5
Manage Your Time

Stress can often stem from feeling overwhelmed or overcommitted. Consider prioritizing your tasks and setting realistic goals to reduce stress and increase productivity.

Tip 6
Practice Relaxation Techniques

Relaxation techniques, such as deep breathing, progressive muscle relaxation, and guided imagery, can help reduce stress and promote relaxation.

Tip 6
Seek Professional Help

If stress is affecting your weight loss efforts and overall health, consider seeking professional help. A therapist or counselor can help you develop effective stress management strategies and support you in your weight loss journey.

TECHNIQUES FOR MANAGING STRESS

Stress is an inevitable part of life and can have a significant impact on both our mental and physical well-being. When it comes to weight loss, stress can have a detrimental effect, causing us to turn to unhealthy coping mechanisms such as overeating or skipping physical activity. Fortunately, there are several effective techniques that can help us manage stress and maintain a healthy weight.

Exercise: Exercise is a great way to reduce stress and improve mental health. Physical activity releases endorphins, which are natural mood enhancers that can reduce feelings of anxiety and depression. Additionally, exercise provides a healthy outlet for pent-up energy and frustration, helping to reduce overall stress levels.

Mindfulness and Meditation: Practicing mindfulness and meditation can help us to focus on the present moment and reduce feelings of anxiety and stress. Mindfulness meditation involves paying attention to the present moment without judgment, while deep breathing exercises can also help to calm the mind and reduce stress.

Time Management: Effective time management can help to reduce stress by preventing us from feeling overwhelmed and overworked. This can be achieved by prioritizing tasks, setting realistic deadlines, and learning to say "no" to unnecessary commitments.

Relaxation Techniques: Relaxation techniques such as yoga, tai chi, and progressive muscle relaxation can help to reduce stress and improve overall mental health. These techniques involve specific exercises that help to calm the mind and reduce physical tension, leading to a more relaxed and stress-free state.

Social Support: Having a strong support system can be crucial in managing stress and reducing its impact on our mental and physical well-being. Talking to friends and family, participating in social activities, and seeking support from a therapist or counselor can help to reduce feelings of isolation and increase feelings of support and connection.

Sleep: Getting enough sleep is essential for managing stress and improving overall health. Lack of sleep can lead to increased stress and irritability, making it more difficult to cope with life's challenges. Aiming for 7-9 hours of sleep each night can help to reduce stress and improve overall well-being.

Healthy Eating: Eating a balanced and nutritious diet can help to reduce stress by providing the body with the nutrients it needs to function properly. Consuming foods high in vitamins and minerals, such as fruits and vegetables, can help to boost the immune system and reduce feelings of stress and anxiety.

Humor and Laughter: Laughter can be an excellent

way to reduce stress and improve overall mental health. Engaging in activities that bring joy and laughter, such as watching a funny movie or reading a humorous book, can help to reduce feelings of stress and improve mood.

Nature: Spending time in nature can help to reduce stress and improve overall mental health. Studies have shown that exposure to nature can reduce feelings of anxiety, depression, and stress, and improve overall well-being.

In conclusion, stress can have a significant impact on weight loss and overall health, but with the right techniques and tools, it can be effectively managed. From exercise and mindfulness meditation to social support and healthy eating, there are many effective techniques that can help us reduce stress and maintain a healthy weight. The key is to find the techniques that work best for you and make them a part of your daily routine. With the right tools and support, you can achieve your weight loss goals and live a healthier, happier life.

IMPORTANCE OF SLEEP FOR WEIGHT LOSS

Sleep plays a crucial role in overall health and wellness, including weight loss. While diet and exercise are important for managing weight, getting enough sleep is also crucial for success. The link between sleep and weight loss is complex, but several factors make sleep an important consideration for people who want to lose weight and maintain a healthy weight.

When we don't get enough sleep, our bodies experience changes that can make it more difficult to lose weight. Lack of sleep has been linked to hormonal imbalances that increase appetite and cravings for high-calorie, sugary foods. This is because lack of sleep leads to an increase in the hunger hormone ghrelin and a decrease in the hormone leptin, which regulates feelings of fullness. When we don't get enough sleep, our bodies become less sensitive to insulin, making it harder for us to control our blood sugar levels and leading to increased food cravings.

Sleep also affects our metabolism. Studies have shown that people who get less sleep tend to have a slower metabolism than those who get enough sleep. This means that their bodies burn fewer calories even when they are resting, making it more difficult to lose weight. Lack of sleep also affects the body's ability to store and use energy efficiently, making it more difficult to lose weight and keep it off.

In addition to the hormonal and metabolic effects of sleep, lack of sleep can also have a negative impact on our physical activity levels. People who don't get enough sleep tend to have less energy and feel more fatigued, making it harder for them to engage in regular physical activity. This can further impact weight loss, as physical activity is a key component of a healthy weight management plan.

In order to maximize the impact of sleep on weight loss, it is recommended that adults get 7-9 hours of sleep per night. However, the amount of sleep that is right for you may vary based on your individual needs. To determine the amount of sleep you need, pay attention to how you feel during the day. If you feel tired and sluggish, you may need to get more sleep. If you feel energized and alert, you are likely getting enough sleep.

Sleep quality is just as important as the amount of sleep you get. To improve the quality of your sleep, consider implementing the following strategies:

Establish a consistent sleep schedule. Try to go to bed and wake up at the same time every day, even on weekends. This will help regulate your circadian rhythm and improve the quality of your sleep.

Create a sleep-conducive environment. Make sure your sleep environment is cool, dark, and quiet. Use curtains or blinds to block out light, and consider using a white noise machine to reduce noise levels.

Limit caffeine and alcohol. Both caffeine and alcohol can affect the quality of your sleep, so it's best to avoid them in the hours leading up to bedtime.

Relax before bed. Taking a warm bath, practicing deep breathing exercises, or reading a book can help you relax and prepare for sleep.

Avoid screens before bedtime. The blue light emitted by screens can interfere with your circadian rhythm, making it harder to fall asleep. Try to avoid screens for at least an hour before bedtime.

Get physical activity during the day. Regular physical activity can improve the quality of your sleep and help you fall asleep more easily at night.

Getting enough sleep is an important part of a comprehensive weight loss plan. By prioritizing sleep and implementing strategies to improve the quality of your sleep, you can increase your chances of success and improve your overall health and well-being.

Sleep is an essential aspect of a healthy lifestyle, and it plays a critical role in weight loss. The relationship between sleep and weight loss is complex, with sleep affecting hormones and metabolism, which can impact appetite, food choices, and physical activity levels. In turn, sleep can be impacted by diet, exercise, stress, and other lifestyle factors.

The link between sleep and weight loss

Sleep is crucial for the regulation of hormones that control hunger and metabolism. Leptin and ghrelin are two hormones that play a key role in regulating appetite.

Leptin is known as the "satiety hormone," as it signals the brain when you have eaten enough and suppresses appetite.

Ghrelin, on the other hand, is known as the "hunger hormone," as it stimulates appetite and increases food cravings. When you are sleep-deprived, levels of leptin decrease, while levels of ghrelin increase, leading to increased hunger and cravings. This can result in overeating and weight gain.

In addition to hormonal regulation, sleep can also impact your metabolism.The National Sleep Foundation reports that sleep deprivation can slow down the metabolism, reducing the number of calories burned throughout the day. This, combined with increased hunger, can make it more challenging to maintain a healthy weight.

Moreover, sleep and physical activity are interconnected. When you are tired, you are less likely to engage in physical activity, and you may have less energy for physical activity. This can negatively impact weight loss, as physical activity is a crucial component of a healthy weight loss program.

IMPROVING YOUR SLEEP HABITS

Establish a regular sleep routine

One of the most important things you can do to improve your sleep is to establish a regular sleep routine. Go to bed and wake up at the same time every day, even on weekends, to help regulate your circadian rhythm. This will make it easier for you to fall asleep and wake up feeling refreshed.

Create a sleep-conducive environment

Your sleep environment can greatly impact your ability to fall asleep and stay asleep. Make sure your bedroom is quiet, cool, and dark. Reduce noise, light, and electronic distractions, such as televisions and phones, in your bedroom. If necessary, invest in earplugs, blackout curtains, or a white noise machine to create a peaceful sleep environment.

Limit caffeine and alcohol

Caffeine and alcohol can disrupt sleep, making it more challenging to fall asleep and stay asleep. Limit caffeine consumption to the morning and early afternoon and avoid alcohol before bedtime. If you are having trouble sleeping, consider cutting out caffeine and alcohol altogether.

Engage in relaxation techniques before bed

Relaxation techniques, such as deep breathing, meditation, and yoga, can help you wind down and prepare for sleep. Find a relaxation technique that works for you and incorporate it into your pre-sleep routine. This can help you calm your mind and fall asleep more quickly.

Limit late-night snacking

Eating late at night can disrupt your sleep, causing discomfort and indigestion. To promote better sleep, limit late-night snacking and eat your last meal at least two hours before bedtime.

Get regular physical activity

Physical activity can help improve the quality of your sleep and make it easier to fall asleep. Engage in regular physical activity, but avoid strenuous exercise close to bedtime, as this can make it more challenging to fall asleep.

CHAPTER FIVE

STRATEGY 4

STAYING MOTIVATED AND ON TRACK

SETTING REALISTIC GOAL

Setting realistic weight loss goals is a crucial step in achieving long-term success in your weight loss journey.

A well-defined goal can serve as a roadmap, providing direction and motivation, while also keeping you accountable. But it's important to understand that not all goals are created equal. Unrealistic goals can be discouraging and even demotivating, leading to frustration and a lack of progress. In order to set effective weight loss goals, it's important to understand the following:

Your starting point: Before setting your weight loss goal, it's important to determine your starting point. This includes your current weight, body composition, and other relevant health metrics. Understanding where you are starting from will give you a baseline to work from and help you set realistic goals.

Your weight loss rate: The rate at which you can realistically lose weight depends on a variety of factors, including your starting weight, diet, exercise routine, and metabolism. It's important to keep in mind that a safe and healthy rate of weight loss is typically 1-2 pounds per week.

Your body composition: Body composition refers to the proportion of fat and muscle in your body. As you lose weight, it's important to keep in mind that muscle mass may decrease along with fat mass. This is why it's important to focus on both weight loss and body composition goals.

Your lifestyle: Your lifestyle and daily habits play a major role in your ability to lose weight and keep it off. It's important to consider the impact of your daily routines and habits on your weight loss goals. For example, if you have a sedentary job and don't exercise regularly, it may be more challenging to lose weight than if you are physically active.

With these considerations in mind, you can set realistic weight loss goals that are both achievable and

sustainable. Here are some tips to help you get started:

- Be specific: Specify a target weight, body composition, or other relevant metric that you want to achieve. The more specific your goal, the easier it will be to track progress and stay motivated.

- Make it measurable: Make your goal measurable by setting a deadline for when you want to achieve it. This will give you a sense of urgency and help keep you on track.

- Set intermediate goals: Break your larger goal into smaller, intermediate goals. This can help you see progress along the way and stay motivated.

- Make it attainable: Ensure that your goal is attainable by considering your starting point, weight loss rate, body composition, and lifestyle.

- Make it relevant: Make your goal relevant to your life and values. For example, if you value being healthy and active, make that the focus of your weight loss goal.

- Make it time-bound: Set a deadline for when you want to achieve your goal. This will give you a sense of urgency and help keep you on track.

By following these guidelines, you can set realistic weight loss goals that are achievable, sustainable, and motivating. Remember that progress takes time, so be patient with yourself and celebrate each small victory along the way. With a clear roadmap and a commitment to making healthy lifestyle changes, you can reach your weight loss goals and achieve the healthy, active life you deserve.

BUILDING A SUPPORT SYSTEM

Building a support system is an essential aspect of effective weight loss. When it comes to losing weight, it is important to have a solid support system in place to help you overcome obstacles and stay motivated. A supportive network can provide the encouragement, accountability, and emotional support necessary to reach your weight loss goals.

One of the first steps in building a support system is to identify the people in your life who are most likely to support you. This may include family members, friends, coworkers, or members of a support group. Once you have identified your support network, it is important to communicate your goals and ask for their support.

One of the biggest benefits of having a supportive network is accountability. When you have people in your life who are aware of your weight loss goals, you are more likely to stay on track and avoid falling back into old habits. For example, if you know that you have a workout buddy who is counting on you to show up at the gym, you are more likely to make exercise a priority. Additionally, having someone to share your progress with can provide a sense of accomplishment and help keep you motivated.

Another benefit of having a support system is emotional support. Losing weight can be a challenging and emotional journey, and it is important to have people in your life who understand and support your goals. This can include people who have gone through a similar experience or who simply understand the importance of a healthy lifestyle. Having someone to turn to during difficult times can make all the difference in staying committed to your weight loss goals.

It is also important to be aware of the emotional impact of weight loss. Losing weight can bring up a range of emotions, including excitement, fear, guilt, and sadness. For some, it can be difficult to reconcile the body they see in the mirror with the image they have of themselves. It is important to have a support system in place to help you process these emotions and overcome any feelings of discouragement or doubt.

Building a support system can take time and effort, but the benefits are well worth it. There are a variety of ways to build a support system, including:

- Joining a support group: This can be an excellent way to connect with others who are going through similar experiences. Support groups can provide a sense of community and offer a safe space to share your struggles and triumphs.

- Relying on a workout buddy: Having a workout buddy can be a great way to stay accountable and stay motivated. It can also be a fun way to bond with a friend and get some exercise in the process.

- Connecting with a coach or mentor: A coach or mentor can provide you with guidance and support as you navigate your weight loss journey. They can also offer tips and advice on how to overcome challenges and stay committed to your goals.

- Utilizing online resources: There are a variety of online resources available for those looking to lose weight. This can include websites, forums, and social media groups that offer support, information, and resources for those seeking to improve their health.

- In conclusion, building a supportive network is an essential aspect of effective weight loss. Having people in your life who understand and support your goals can provide the accountability, emotional support, and motivation necessary to achieve your weight loss goals. Whether it's a workout buddy, a support group, or a coach, having a solid support system in place can help you overcome obstacles and reach your goals

OVERCOMING PLATEAUS AND SETBACKS IN YOUR WEIGHT LOSS JOURNEY

a. Losing weight can be a challenging and often frustrating journey, and one of the biggest obstacles is hitting a plateau or experiencing setbacks. However, it's important to remember that setbacks are a normal part of the process and can actually help you grow stronger and become more committed to your goals. Here are some tips for overcoming plateaus and setbacks in your weight loss journey:

b. Assess your habits: It's possible that your weight loss has plateaued because you've fallen into bad habits, such as eating too many processed foods or not getting enough exercise. Take a step back and assess your habits, both good and bad, to identify areas for improvement.

c. Track your progress: Tracking your progress can help you identify patterns and trends in your weight loss journey. This information can be used to identify what's working and what's not, allowing you to make adjustments as needed.

d. Get more active: Increasing your physical activity is one of the best ways to overcome a weight loss plateau. Adding more exercise to your routine can help increase your metabolism and burn more calories, which can jumpstart your weight loss.

e. Mix it up: Doing the same workout every day can lead to boredom and a plateau. Mix up your routine by trying new activities, changing the intensity, or working out at different times of the day. This will not only keep things interesting, but it can also help you avoid hitting a plateau.

f. Get support: Surrounding yourself with a supportive network of friends and family can help you stay motivated and on track. Join a weight loss support group, work with a personal trainer, or simply find a workout buddy to help you stay accountable.

g. Be patient: Weight loss is a journey, not a destination. It's important to be patient and give your body time to adjust. Remember that slow and steady progress is better than no progress at all.

h. Don't give up: Finally, it's important to remember that setbacks are a normal part of the process. Don't let a setback discourage you or make you feel like giving up. Instead, use it as an opportunity to reflect, make adjustments, and recommit to your goals.

Hitting a plateau or experiencing a setback in your weight loss journey can be disheartening, but it doesn't have to mean the end of your journey. By assessing your habits, tracking your progress, getting more active, mixing up your routine, getting support, being patient, and not giving up, you can overcome any obstacle and achieve your weight loss goals

CELEBRATING YOUR PROGRESS AND ACCOMPLISHMENTS: THE KEY TO SUSTAINING YOUR WEIGHT LOSS GOALS

Weight loss can be a challenging journey, but it is also a journey of self-discovery, growth, and accomplishment. As you work towards your weight loss goals, it is important to take the time to celebrate your progress and accomplishments. Celebrating your success can help keep you motivated and encourage you to continue making healthy choices.

Here are some ways to celebrate your weight loss progress and accomplishments:

- Keep a journal: Write down your weight loss milestones and your feelings about them. This will not only help you keep track of your progress, but it will also allow you to look back and reflect on your journey. You can also write down what you have learned about yourself and your eating habits and how you have changed as a result of your weight loss journey.

- Reward yourself: Treat yourself to something you have been wanting. This could be something as simple as a new outfit, a spa day, or a special meal. Make sure that your reward is something that will not sabotage your weight loss progress.

- Share your accomplishments: Share your weight loss milestones with your friends, family, and support system. Not only will this help keep you accountable, but it will also help you build a support system. Your loved ones will be proud of your progress and will help keep you motivated.

- Get involved in a community: Join a weight loss support group or a fitness community. You will be able to connect with others who are on a similar journey, and you can share your successes and struggles. You will also have the opportunity to learn from others and gain inspiration from their progress.

- Take photos: Document your progress by taking photos. You can see your progress in a tangible way and it will help you stay motivated. It's also fun to look back on old photos and see how far you have come.

- Celebrate non-scale victories: Celebrate milestones like fitting into a pair of jeans that were too tight, running a mile without stopping, or completing a fitness class. These non-scale victories are just as important as the numbers on the scale and should be celebrated just as much.

- Practice gratitude: Take time to appreciate all the

positive changes in your life that have resulted from your weight loss journey. This could be improved health, increased energy levels, or a boost in self-esteem. Focusing on the positive changes in your life can help keep you motivated.

- Celebrating your progress and accomplishments is a key factor in maintaining your weight loss goals. It helps you stay motivated, keep your spirits high, and feel good about your progress. By recognizing and celebrating your successes, you will be more likely to continue making healthy choices and reaching your weight loss goals.

In conclusion, weight loss is not just about losing weight, it's about making a commitment to yourself to live a healthier and happier life. Celebrating your progress and accomplishments is a way to acknowledge the hard work and effort you have put into your journey. So, take the time to celebrate your successes, no matter how big or small, and enjoy the journey.

CHAPTER SIX

FINAL THOUGHTS ON EFFECTIVE WEIGHT LOSS GOALS

Losing weight can be a challenging journey, but it can also be one of the most rewarding experiences of your life. By setting realistic goals, developing a healthy diet, engaging in regular physical activity, managing stress and sleep habits, and building a supportive network, you can achieve your weight loss goals and maintain a healthy weight for life.

It is important to remember that weight loss is not a one-size-fits-all process and that everyone's journey is unique. Some people may see results quickly, while others may take longer to reach their goals. It is also important to understand that weight loss is not just about reaching a specific number on the scale, but also about improving your overall health and well-being.

One of the keys to effective weight loss is making lasting lifestyle changes, rather than just trying quick fixes or fad diets. This means incorporating healthy eating habits, regular physical activity, stress management techniques, and quality sleep into your daily routine. It may take time and effort, but the results will be worth it in the end.

Another important aspect of effective weight loss is staying motivated and celebrating your progress and accomplishments along the way. This can be as simple as keeping a journal or food diary to track your progress, or setting achievable milestones and rewarding yourself when you reach them.

It is also important to be kind to yourself and not beat yourself up over setbacks or plateaus. Weight loss is not always a linear process, and there may be times when you feel like you're not making progress. It is important to keep a positive outlook and focus on the progress you have made, rather than dwelling on setbacks.

Next Steps To Achieving Your Weight Loss Goals

- Losing weight can be a journey filled with ups and downs, but with determination and perseverance, you can achieve your weight loss goals. Here are some steps you can take to ensure success:

- Reevaluate your goals: Take a moment to reflect on your weight loss goals and ensure that they are still realistic and achievable. If necessary, adjust your goals to reflect your current lifestyle and circumstances.

- Create a plan: Once you have set your weight loss goals, create a plan to achieve them. This may include incorporating healthier eating habits, engaging in regular physical activity, managing stress, and improving your sleep habits.

- Stay accountable: Keeping a journal or food diary can help you stay accountable and track your progress. Consider working with a dietician or fitness coach who can provide guidance and support along the way.

- Stay active: Regular physical activity is an important aspect of weight loss. Incorporate physical activity into your daily routine, whether it's taking a walk, joining a gym, or participating in a sports team.

- Focus on healthy eating habits: Adopting healthy eating habits, such as eating more fruits and vegetables, reducing processed foods, and managing portion sizes, can help you reach your weight loss goals.

- Manage stress: Stress can impact weight loss, so it is important to find healthy ways to manage it, such as practicing meditation, yoga, or deep breathing exercises.

- Get enough sleep: Adequate sleep is crucial for weight loss, as it can help regulate hormones and improve energy levels. Aim for 7-9 hours of sleep each night.

- Surround yourself with support: Building a

supportive network of friends and family members who encourage and motivate you can be an invaluable resource as you work to achieve your weight loss goals.

- Celebrate your progress: Celebrate your progress and accomplishments along the way, whether it's reaching a milestone or simply feeling proud of your hard work and dedication.

- Be patient: Weight loss is a journey and not a quick fix. Be patient and kind to yourself as you work towards your goals.

Books and Articles on Weight Loss

"The Complete Guide to Fat Loss" by Dr. Arjun Das

"The Ultimate Guide to Weight Loss" by Dr. Michael Mosley and Mimi Spencer

"The 4-Hour Body" by Tim Ferriss

"The Weight Loss Cure 'They' Don't Want You to Know About" by Kevin Trudeau

"The Beck Diet Solution: Train Your Brain to Think Like

a Thin Person" by Judith Beck

"The Diet Fix: Why Diets Fail and How to Make Yours Work" by Yoni Freedhoff, M.D.

"The New Rules of Lifting for Women: Lift Like a Man, Look Like a Goddess" by Lou Schuler and Cassandra Forsythe

"Mindless Eating: Why We Eat More Than We Think" by Brian Wansink

"The Complete Idiot's Guide to Weight Loss" by Dr. Deirdre Rawlings

"The Weight Loss Diaries" by Ted Spiker

Websites and Online Resources for Healthy Living:

MyFitnessPal

LoseIt!

SparkPeople

Noom

MyPlate by Livestrong

caloriecount.com

EatingWell

Shape

Healthline

How to loss weight fast.

WebMD

---

¹ How to loss weight fast: 4 strategy to effective weight loss in 7 days

ABOUT THE AUTHOR

Celestine Benedict is a passionate health and wellness writer with a focus on weight loss. With years of experience in the field, he has a wealth of knowledge and expertise that he brings to his writing. His passion for helping others achieve their health and wellness goals has driven him to share his insights and advice with the world through his writing.

As a health and wellness enthusiast, [Your Name] has dedicated his life to researching and learning about the latest and most effective methods for weight loss. He has a deep understanding of the complexities and challenges associated with weight loss, and he is committed to providing his readers with practical, actionable, and evidence-based advice.

He takes a holistic approach to health and wellness, incorporating both physical and mental health into his recommendations. He recognizes that weight loss is a journey that requires commitment, discipline, and patience, and he is dedicated to providing his readers with the tools and guidance they need to succeed.